CW00552027

The Ultimate Keto Vegetarian Cookbook for Busy People

Enjoy A Collection of Tasty and Healthy Keto Vegan for Dessert Lovers

Skye Webb

DESSERTS

Table of contents

Maple-Walnut Oatmeal Cookies

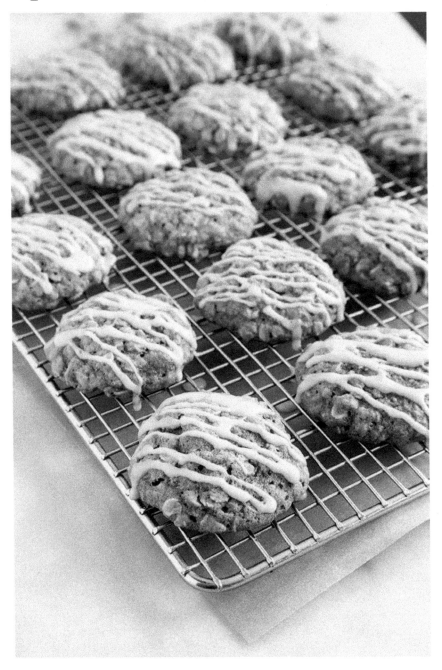

Preparation time: 5 minutes cooking time: 10 minutes servings: about 2 dozen cookies

Ingredients

1½ cups whole-grain flour

1 teaspoon baking powder

⅛ teaspoon salt

1   teaspoon ground cinnamon

¼ teaspoon ground nutmeg

1½ cups old-fashioned oats

1 cup chopped walnuts

½ cup vegan margarine, melted

½ cup pure maple syrup

¼ cup light brown sugar

2   teaspoons pure vanilla extract

Directions

1.   Preheat the oven to 375°F. In a large bowl, sift together the flour, baking powder, salt, cinnamon, and nutmeg. Stir in the oats and walnuts.

2.   In a medium bowl, combine the margarine, maple syrup, sugar, and vanilla and mix well.

3.   Add the wet Ingredients to the dry Ingredients, stirring to mix well.

4.   Drop the cookie dough by the tablespoonful onto an ungreased baking sheet and press down slightly with a fork. Bake until browned, 10 to 12 minutes. Cool the cookies slightly before transferring to a wire rack to cool completely. Store in an airtight container.

Banana-Nut Bread Bars

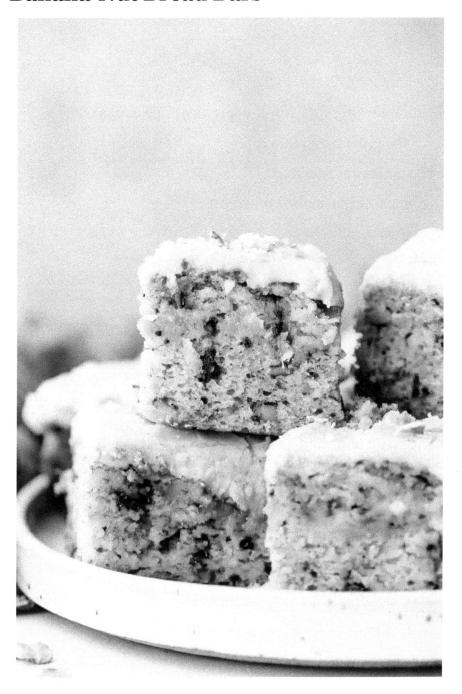

Preparation time: 5 minutes cooking time: 30 minutes

servings: 9 bars

Ingredients

Nonstick cooking spray (optional 2 large ripe bananas

1   tablespoon maple syrup

½ teaspoon vanilla extract

2   cups old-fashioned rolled oats

½ teaspoons salt

¼ cup chopped walnuts

Directions

1.   Preheat the oven to 350°F. Lightly coat a 9-by-9-inch baking pan with nonstick cooking spray (if usingor line with parchment paper for oil-free baking.

2.   In a medium bowl, mash the bananas with a fork. Add the maple syrup and vanilla extract and mix well. Add the oats, salt, and walnuts, mixing well.

3.   Transfer the batter to the baking pan and bake for 25 to 30 minutes, until the top is crispy. Cool completely before slicing into 9 bars. Transfer to an airtight storage container or a large plastic bag.

Nutrition (1 bar): Calories: 73; Fat: 1g; Protein: 2g; Carbohydrates: 15g; Fiber: 2g; Sugar: 5g; Sodium: 129mg

Apple Crumble

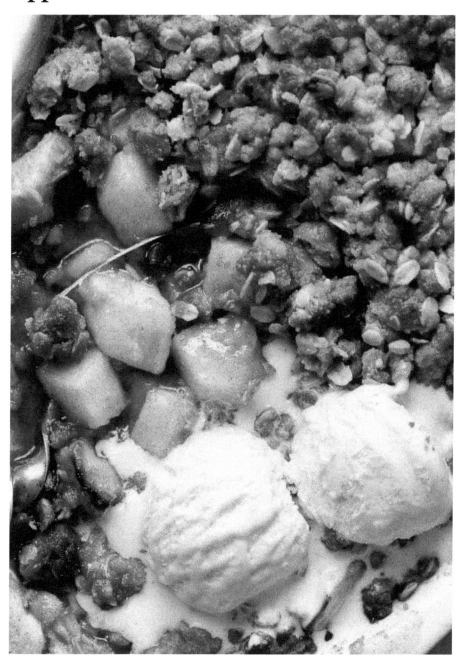

Preparation time: 20 minutes cooking time: 25 minutes servings: 6

Ingredients For the filling

4 to 5 apples, cored and chopped (about 6 cups

½ cup unsweetened applesauce, or ¼ cup water

2 to 3 tablespoons unrefined sugar (coconut, date, sucanat, maple syrup 1 teaspoon ground cinnamon

Pinch sea salt

For the crumble

2 tablespoons almond butter, or cashew or sunflower seed butter 2 tablespoons maple syrup

1½ cups rolled oats

½ cup walnuts, finely chopped

½ teaspoon ground cinnamon

2 to 3 tablespoons unrefined granular sugar (coconut, date, sucanat

Directions

1.   Preheat the oven to 350°F. Put the apples and applesauce in an 8-inch-square baking dish, and sprinkle with the sugar, cinnamon, and salt. Toss to combine.

2.   In a medium bowl, mix together the nut butter and maple syrup until smooth and creamy. Add the oats, walnuts, cinnamon, and sugar and stir to coat, using your hands if necessary. (If you

have a small food processor, pulse the oats and walnuts together before adding them to the mix.

3.   Sprinkle the topping over the apples, and put the dish in the oven.

4.   Bake for 20 to 25 minutes, or until the fruit is soft and the topping is lightly browned.

Nutrition Calories: 356; Total fat: 17g; Carbs: 49g; Fiber: 7g; Protein: 7g

Chocolate-Cranberry Oatmeal Cookies

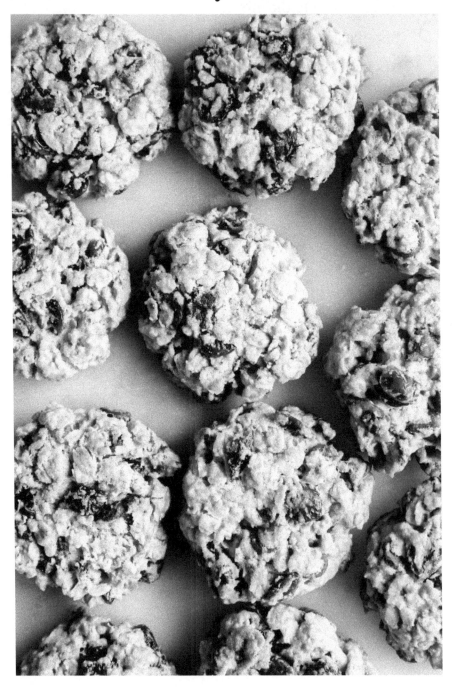

Preparation time: 5 minutes cooking time: 15 minutes servings: about 2 dozen cookies

Ingredients

½ cup vegan margarine

1 cup sugar

¼ cup apple juice

1 cup whole-grain flour

1 teaspoon baking powder

½ teaspoon salt

1 teaspoon pure vanilla extract

1 cup old-fashioned oats

½ cup vegan semisweet chocolate chips

½ cup sweetened dried cranberries

Directions

1.　　Preheat the oven to 375°F. In a large bowl, cream together the margarine and the sugar until light and fluffy. Blend in the juice.

2.　　Add the flour, baking powder, salt, and vanilla, blending well. Stir in the oats, chocolate chips, and cranberries and mix well.

3.　　Drop the dough from a teaspoon onto an ungreased baking sheet. Bake until nicely browned, about 15

 minutes. Cool the cookies slightly before transferring to a wire rack to cool completely. Store in an airtight container.

Cashew-Chocolate Truffles

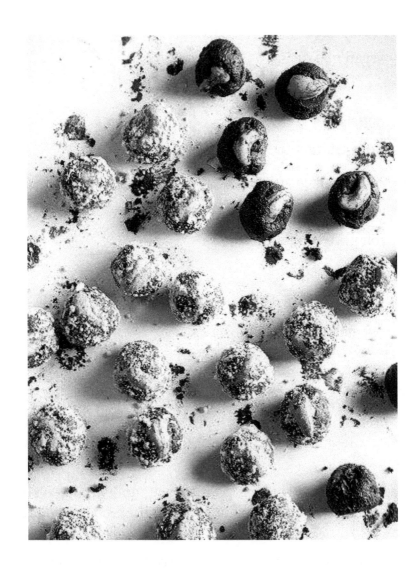

Preparation time: 15 minutes

cooking time: 0 minutes • plus 1 hour to set servings: 12 truffles

Ingredients

1   cup raw cashews, soaked in water overnight

¾ cup pitted dates

2   tablespoons coconut oil

1 cup unsweetened shredded coconut, divided 1 to 2 tablespoons

cocoa powder, to taste

Directions

1.   In a food processor, combine the cashews, dates, coconut oil, ½ cup of shredded coconut, and cocoa powder. Pulse until fully incorporated; it will resemble chunky cookie dough. Spread the remaining ½ cup of shredded coconut on a plate.

2.   Form the mixture into tablespoon-size balls and roll on the plate to cover with the shredded coconut. Transfer to a parchment paper–lined plate or baking sheet. Repeat to make 12 truffles.

3.   Place the truffles in the refrigerator for 1 hour to set. Transfer the truffles to a storage container or freezer-safe bag and seal.

Nutrition (1 truffle): Calories 238: Fat: 18g; Protein: 3g; Carbohydrates: 16g; Fiber: 4g; Sugar: 9g; Sodium: 9mg

Banana Chocolate Cupcakes

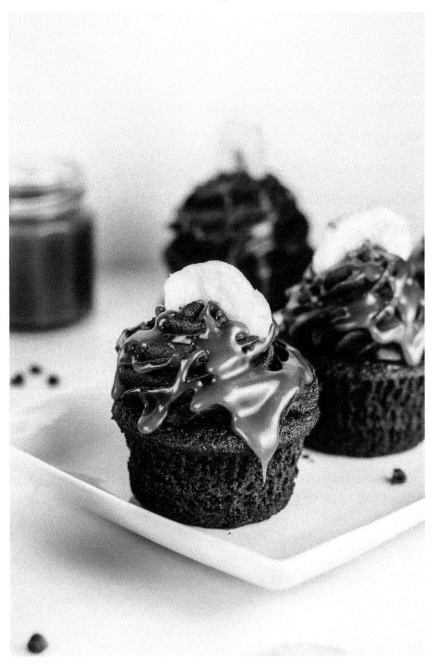

Preparation time: 20 minutes cooking time: 20 minutes servings: 12 cupcakes

Ingredients

3 medium bananas

1   cup non-dairy milk

2   tablespoons almond butter

1   teaspoon apple cider vinegar

1 teaspoon pure vanilla extract 1¼ cups whole-wheat flour

½ cup rolled oats

¼ cup coconut sugar (optional 1 teaspoon baking powder

½ teaspoon baking soda

½ cup unsweetened cocoa powder

¼ cup chia seeds, or sesame seeds

Pinch sea salt

¼ cup dark chocolate chips, dried cranberries, or raisins (optional

Directions

1.   Preheat the oven to 350°F. Lightly grease the cups of two 6-cup muffin tins or line with paper muffin cups.

2.   Put the bananas, milk, almond butter, vinegar, and vanilla in a blender and purée until smooth. Or stir together in a large bowl until smooth and creamy.

3.   Put the flour, oats, sugar (if using), baking powder, baking soda, cocoa powder, chia seeds, salt, and chocolate chips in another large bowl, and stir to combine. Mix together the wet and dry ingredients,

stirring as little as possible. Spoon into muffin cups, and bake for 20 to 25 minutes. Take the cupcakes out of the oven and let them cool fully before taking out of the muffin tins, since they'll be very moist.

Nutrition (1 cupcakeCalories: 215; Total fat: 6g; Carbs: 39g; Fiber: 9g; Protein: 6g

Minty Fruit Salad

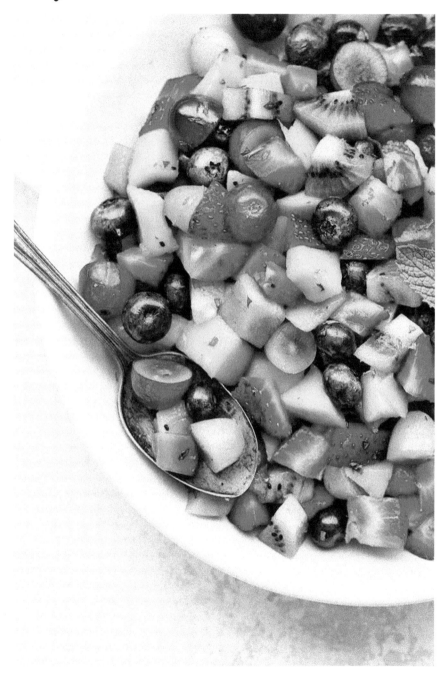

Preparation time: 15 minutes cooking time: 5 minutes servings: 4

Ingredients

¼ cup lemon juice (about 2 small lemons 4 teaspoons maple syrup or agave syrup

2 cups chopped pineapple

2   cups chopped strawberries

2 cups raspberries

1 cup blueberries

8 fresh mint leaves

Directions

1.   Beginning with 1 mason jar, add the ingredients in this order:

2.   1 tablespoon of lemon juice, 1 teaspoon of maple syrup, ½ cup of pineapple, ½ cup of strawberries, ½ cup of raspberries, ¼ cup of blueberries, and 2 mint leaves.

3.   Repeat to fill 3 more jars. Close the jars tightly with lids.

4.   Place the airtight jars in the refrigerator for up to 3 days.

Nutrition: Calories: 138; Fat: 1g; Protein: 2g; Carbohydrates: 34g; Fiber: 8g; Sugar: 22g; Sodium: 6mg

Sesame Cookies

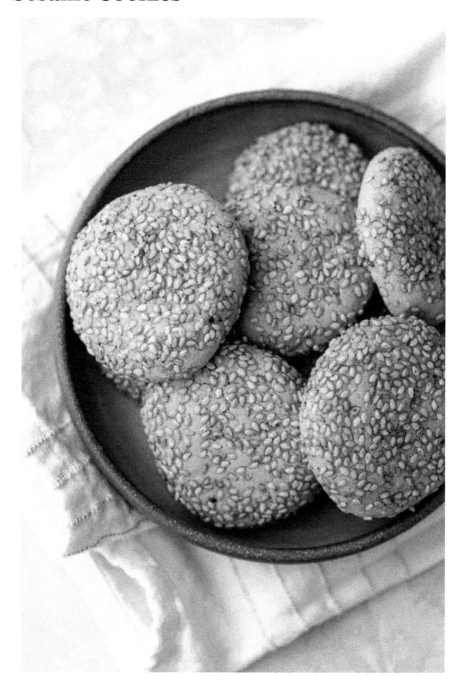

Preparation time: 15 minutes cooking time: 0 minutes servings: 3 dozen cookies

Ingredients

¾ cup vegan margarine, softened

½ cup light brown sugar

1   teaspoon pure vanilla extract

tablespoons pure maple syrup

¼ teaspoon salt

2   cups whole-grain flour

¾ cup sesame seeds, lightly toasted

Directions

1.   In a large bowl, cream together the margarine and sugar until light and fluffy. Blend in the vanilla, maple syrup, and salt. Stir in the flour and sesame seeds and mix well.

2.   Roll the dough into a cylinder about 2 inches in diameter. Wrap it in plastic wrap and refrigerate for 1 hour or longer. Preheat the oven to 325°F.

3.   Slice the cookie dough into 1/8-inch-thick rounds and arrange on an ungreased baking sheet about 2 inches apart. Bake until light brown, about 12 minutes. When completely cool, store in an airtight container.

Mango Coconut Cream Pie

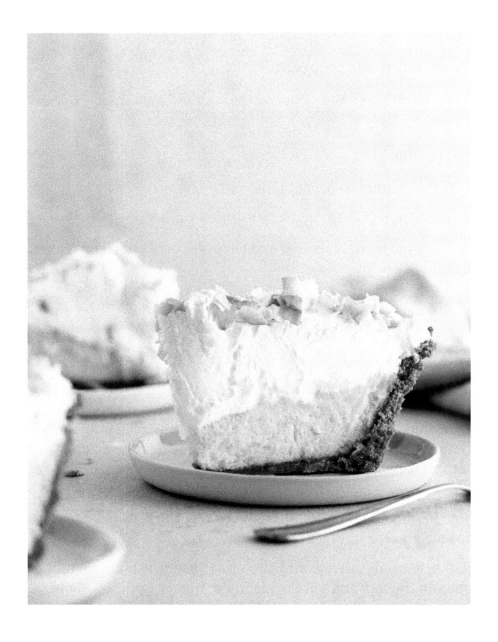

Preparation time: 20 minutes • chill time: 30 minutes servings: 8

Ingredients

For the crust

½ cup rolled oats 1 cup cashews

1 cup soft pitted dates

For the filling

1   cup canned coconut milk

½ cup water

2   large mangos, peeled and chopped, or about 2 cups frozen chunks

½ cup unsweetened shredded coconut

Directions

1.   Put all the crust ingredients in a food processor and pulse until it holds together. If you don't have a food processor, chop everything as finely as possible and use ½ cup cashew or almond butter in place of half the cashews. Press the mixture down firmly into an 8-inch pie or springform pan.

2.   Put the all filling ingredients in a blender and purée until smooth (about 1 minute). It should be very thick, so you may have to stop and stir until it's smooth.

3.   Pour the filling into the crust, use a rubber spatula to smooth the top, and put the pie in the freezer until set, about 30 minutes. Once frozen, it should be set out for about 15 minutes to soften before serving.

4.   Top with a batch of Coconut Whipped Cream scooped on top of the pie once it's set. Finish it off with a sprinkling of toasted shredded coconut.

Nutrition (1 sliceCalories: 427; Total fat: 28g; Carbs: 45g; Fiber: 6g; Protein: 8g

Cherry-Vanilla Rice Pudding (Pressure cooker

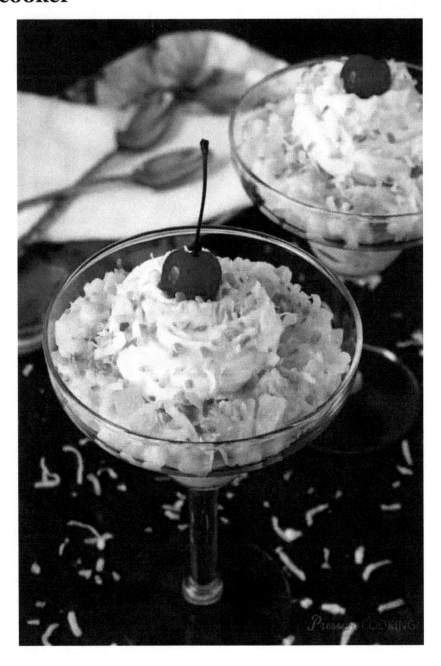

Preparation time: 5 minutes Servings: 4-6

Ingredients

1 cup short-grain brown rice

1¾ cups nondairy milk, plus more as needed

1½ cups water

4 tablespoons unrefined sugar or pure maple syrup (use 2 tablespoons if you use a sweetened milk), plus more as needed

1 teaspoon vanilla extract (use ½ teaspoon if you use vanilla milk Pinch salt

¼ cup dried cherries or ½ cup fresh or frozen pitted cherries

Directions

1.	In your electric pressure cooker's cooking pot, combine the rice, milk, water, sugar, vanilla, and salt.

2.	High pressure for 30 minutes. Close and lock the lid and ensure the pressure valve is sealed, then select High Pressure and set the time for 30 minutes.

3.	Pressure Release. Once the cook time is complete, let the pressure release naturally, about 20 minutes. Once all the pressure has released, carefully unlock and remove the lid. Stir in the cherries and put the lid back on loosely for about 10 minutes. Serve, adding more milk or sugar, as desired.

Nutrition Calories: 177; Total fat: 1g; Protein: 3g; Sodium: 27mg; Fiber: 2g

Chocolate Coconut Brownies

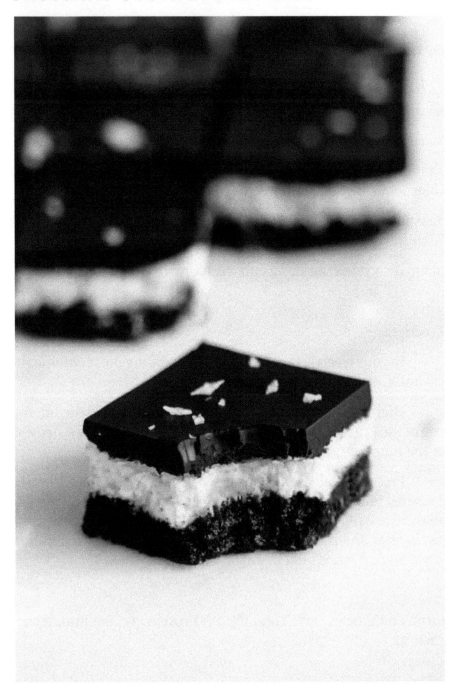

Preparation time: 5 minutes cooking time: 35 minutes servings: 12 brownies

Ingredients

1 cup whole-grain flour

½ cup unsweetened cocoa powder

1 teaspoon baking powder

½ teaspoon salt

1 cup light brown sugar

½ cup canola oil

¾ cup unsweetened coconut milk

1 teaspoon pure vanilla extract

1 teaspoon coconut extract

½ cup vegan semisweet chocolate chips

½ cup sweetened shredded coconut

Directions

1.　　Preheat the oven to 350°F. Grease an 8-inch square baking pan and set aside. In a large bowl, combine the flour, cocoa, baking powder, and salt. Set aside.

2.　　In a medium bowl, mix together the sugar and oil until blended. Stir in the coconut milk

3.　　and the extracts and blend until smooth. Add the wet Ingredients to the dry Ingredients, stirring to blend. Fold in the chocolate chips and coconut.

4.   Scrape the batter into the prepared baking pan and bake until the center is set and a toothpick inserted in the center comes out clean, 35 to 40 minutes. Let the brownies cool 30 minutes before serving. Store in an airtight container.

Lime in the Coconut Chia Pudding

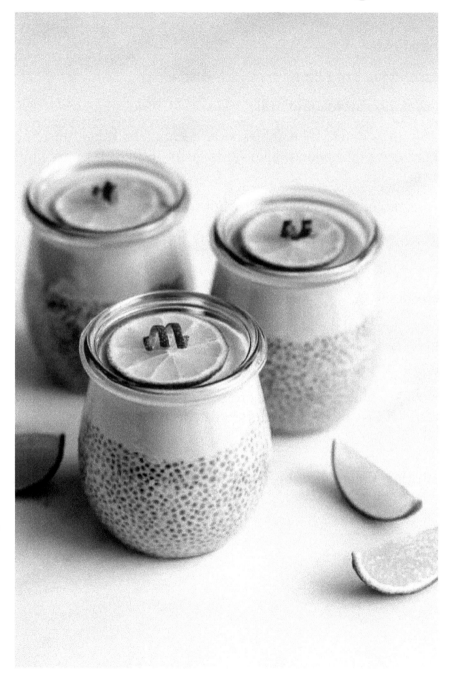

Preparation time: 10 minutes • chill time: 20 minutes servings: 4

Ingredients

Zest and juice of 1 lime

1 (14-ouncecan coconut milk

1   to 2 dates, or 1 tablespoon coconut or other unrefined sugar, or 1 tablespoon maple syrup, or 10 to 15 drops pure liquid stevia

2   tablespoons chia seeds, whole or ground

2 teaspoons matcha green tea powder (optional

Directions

1.   Blend all the ingredients in a blender until smooth. Chill in the fridge for about 20 minutes, then serve topped with one or more of the topping ideas.

2.   Try blueberries, blackberries, sliced strawberries, Coconut Whipped Cream, or toasted unsweetened coconut.

Nutrition Calories: 226; Total fat: 20g; Carbs: 13g; Fiber: 5g; Protein: 3g

Strawberry Parfaits With Cashew Crème

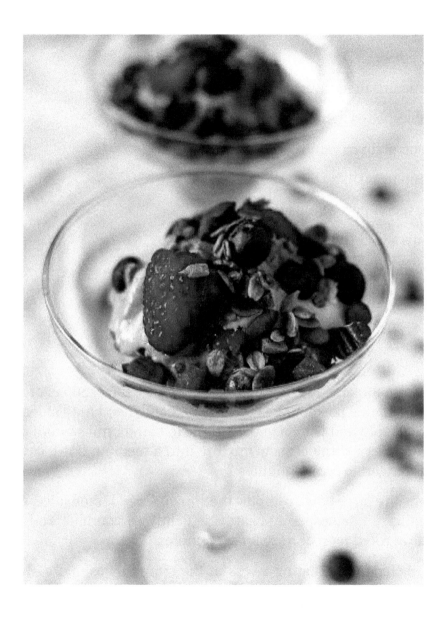

Preparation time: 10 minutes • chill time: 50 minutes • servings: 4

Ingredients

½ cup unsalted raw cashews

4 tablespoons light brown sugar

½ cup plain or vanilla soy milk

¾ cup firm silken tofu, drained

1 teaspoon pure vanilla extract

2 cups sliced strawberries

1 teaspoon fresh lemon juice

Fresh mint leaves, for garnish

Directions

1.   In a blender, grind the cashews and 3 tablespoons of the sugar to a fine powder. Add the soy milk and blend until smooth. Add the tofu and vanilla and continue to blend until smooth and creamy. Scrape the cashew mixture into a medium bowl, cover, and refrigerate for 30 minutes.

2.   In a large bowl, combine the strawberries, lemon juice, and remaining 1 tablespoon sugar. Stir gently to combine and set aside at room temperature for 20 minutes.

3.   Spoon alternating layers of the strawberries and cashew crème into parfait glasses or wineglasses, ending with a dollop of the cashew crème. Garnish with mint leaves and serve.

Mint Chocolate Chip Sorbet

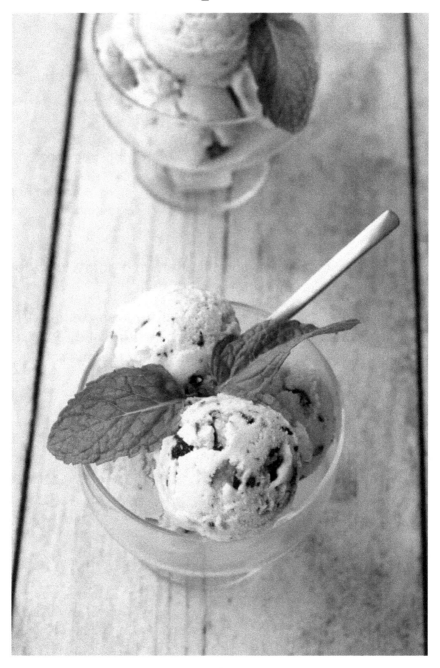

Preparation time: 5 minutes cooking time: 0 minutes servings: 1

Ingredients

1 frozen banana

1   tablespoon almond butter, or peanut butter, or other nut or seed butter 2 tablespoons fresh mint, minced

¼ cup or less non-dairy milk (only if needed

2   to 3 tablespoons non-dairy chocolate chips, or cocoa nibs 2 to 3 tablespoons goji berries (optional

Directions

1.   Put the banana, almond butter, and mint in a food processor or blender and purée until smooth.

2.   Add the non-dairy milk if needed to keep blending (but only if needed, as this will make the texture less solid). Pulse the chocolate chips and goji berries (if usinginto the mix so they're roughly chopped up.

Nutrition Calories: 212; Total fat: 10g; Carbs: 31g; Fiber: 4g; Protein: 3g

Peach-Mango Crumble (Pressure cooker

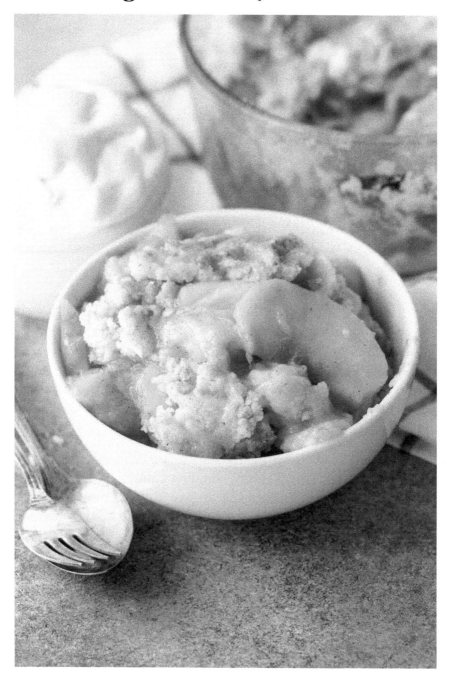

Preparation time: 10 minutes Servings: 4-6

Ingredients

3   cups chopped fresh or frozen peaches

3 cups chopped fresh or frozen mangos

4   tablespoons unrefined sugar or pure maple syrup, divided
1 cup gluten-free rolled oats

½ cup shredded coconut, sweetened or unsweetened

2 tablespoons coconut oil or vegan margarine

Directions

1.   In a 6- to 7-inch round baking dish, toss together the peaches, mangos, and 2 tablespoons of sugar. In a food processor, combine the oats, coconut, coconut oil, and remaining 2 tablespoons of sugar. Pulse until combined. (If you use maple syrup, you'll need less coconut oil. Start with just the syrup and add oil if the mixture isn't sticking together.Sprinkle the oat mixture over the fruit mixture.

2.   Cover the dish with aluminum foil. Put a trivet in the bottom of your electric pressure cooker's cooking pot and pour in a cup or two of water. Using a foil sling or silicone helper handles, lower the pan onto the trivet.

3.   High pressure for 6 minutes. Close and lock the lid and ensure the pressure valve is sealed, then select High Pressure and set the time for 6 minutes.

4.   Pressure Release. Once the cook time is complete, quick release the pressure, being careful not to get your fingers or face near the steam release. Once all the pressure has released, carefully unlock and remove the lid.

5.　　Let cool for a few minutes before carefully lifting out the dish with oven mitts or tongs. Scoop out portions to serve.

Nutrition Calories: 321; Total fat: 18g; Protein: 4g; Sodium: 2mg; Fiber: 7g

Ginger-Spice Brownies

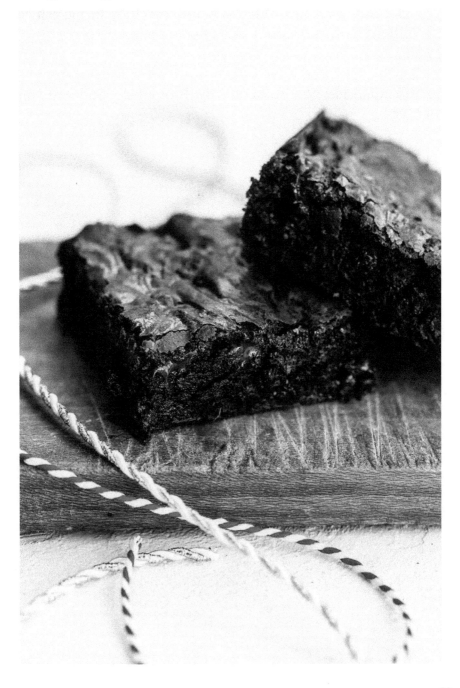

Preparation time: 5 minutes cooking time: 35 minutes servings: 12 brownies

Ingredients

1¾ cups whole-grain flour

1 teaspoon baking powder

1 teaspoon baking soda

½ teaspoon salt

1 tablespoon ground ginger

½ teaspoon ground cinnamon

½ teaspoon ground allspice

3 tablespoons unsweetened cocoa powder

½ cup vegan semisweet chocolate chips

½ cup chopped walnuts

¼ cup canola oil

½ cup dark molasses

½ cup water

⅓ cup light brown sugar

2   teaspoons grated fresh ginger

Directions

1.   Preheat the oven to 350°F. Grease an 8-inch square baking pan and set aside. In a large bowl, combine the flour, baking powder, baking soda, salt, ground ginger, cinnamon, allspice, and cocoa. Stir in the chocolate chips and walnuts and set aside.

2.   In medium bowl, combine the oil, molasses, water, sugar, and fresh ginger and mix well.

3.   Pour the wet Ingredients into the dry Ingredients and mix well.

4.   Scrape the dough into the prepared baking pan. The dough will be sticky, so wet your hands to press it evenly into the pan. Bake until a toothpick inserted in the center comes out clean, 30 to 35 minutes. Cool on a wire rack 30 minutes before cutting. Store in an airtight container.

Chocolate And Walnut Farfalle

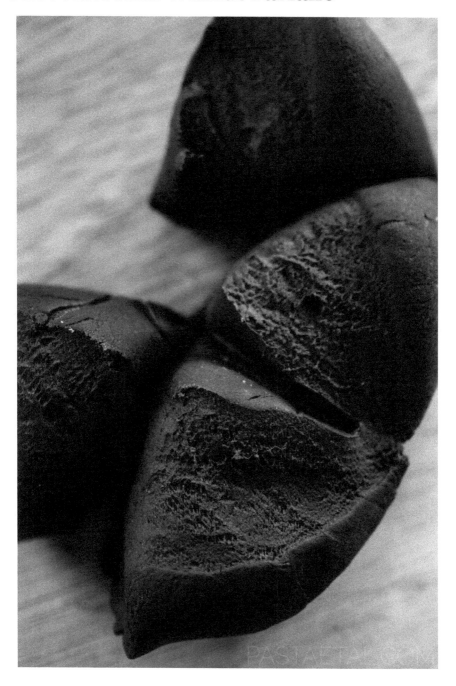

Preparation time: 10 minutes cooking time: 0 minutes servings: 4

Ingredients

½ cup chopped toasted walnuts

¼ cup vegan semisweet chocolate pieces

8 ounces farfalle

3   tablespoons vegan margarine

¼ cup ight brown sugar

Directions

1.   In a food processor or blender, grind the walnuts and chocolate pieces until crumbly. Do not overprocess. Set aside.

2.   In a pot of boiling salted water, cook the farfalle, stirring occasionally, until al dente, about 8 minutes. Drain well and return to the pot.

3.   Add the margarine and sugar and toss to combine and melt the margarine.

4.   Transfer the noodle mixture to a serving

Almond-Date Energy Bites

Preparation time: 5 minutes • chill time: 15 minutes servings: 24 bites

Ingredients

1 cup dates, pitted

1 cup unsweetened shredded coconut

¼ cup chia seeds

¾ cup ground almonds

¼ cup cocoa nibs, or non-dairy chocolate chips

Directions

1.   Purée everything in a food processor until crumbly and sticking together, pushing down the sides whenever necessary to keep it blending. If you don't have a food processor, you can mash soft Medjool dates. But if you're using harder baking dates, you'll have to soak them and then try to purée them in a blender.

2.   Form the mix into 24 balls and place them on a baking sheet lined with parchment or waxed paper. Put in the fridge to set for about 15 minutes. Use the softest dates you can find. Medjool dates are the best for this purpose. The hard dates you see in the baking aisle of your supermarket are going to take a long time to blend up. If you use those, try soaking them in water for at least an hour before you start, and then draining.

Nutrition (1 bite Calories: 152; Total fat: 11g; Carbs: 13g; Fiber: 5g; Protein: 3g

Pumpkin Pie Cups (Pressure cooker)

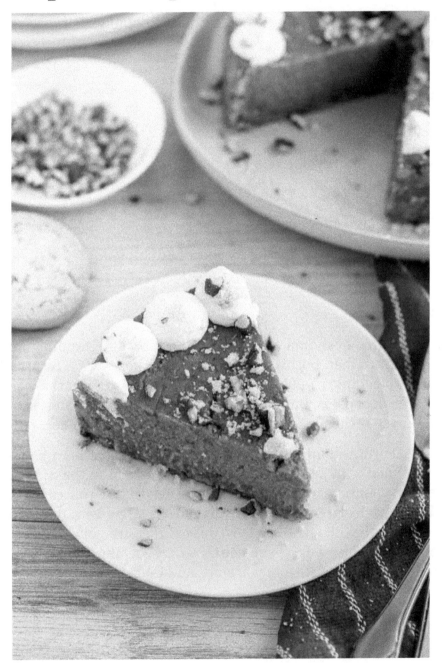

Preparation time: 5 minutes Servings: 4-6

Ingredients

1 cup canned pumpkin purée

1 cup nondairy milk

6 tablespoons unrefined sugar or pure maple syrup (less if using sweetened milk), plus more for sprinkling

¼ cup spelt flour or all-purpose flour

½ teaspoon pumpkin pie spice

Pinch salt

Directions

1.   In a medium bowl, stir together the pumpkin, milk, sugar, flour, pumpkin pie spice, and salt. Pour the mixture into 4 heat-proof ramekins. Sprinkle a bit more sugar on the top of each, if you like. Put a trivet in the bottom of your electric pressure cooker's cooking pot and pour in a cup or two of water. Place the ramekins onto the trivet, stacking them if needed (3 on the bottom, 1 on top).

2.   High pressure for 6 minutes. Close and lock the lid and ensure the pressure valve is sealed, then select High Pressure and set the time for 6 minutes.

3.   Pressure Release. Once the cook time is complete, quick release the pressure, being careful not to get your fingers or face near the steam release. Once all the pressure has released, carefully unlock and remove the lid. Let cool for a few minutes before carefully lifting out the ramekins with oven mitts or tongs. Let cool for at least 10 minutes before serving.

Nutrition Calories: 129; Total fat: 1g; Protein: 3g; Sodium: 39mg; Fiber: 3g

Coconut and Almond Truffles

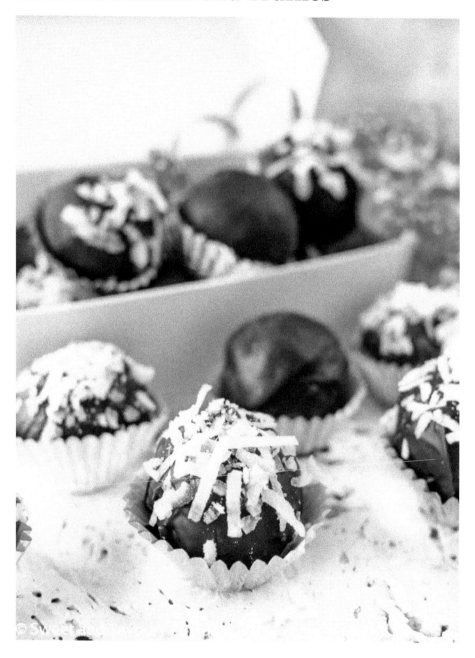

Preparation time: 15 minutes cooking time: 0 minutes servings: 8 truffles

Ingredients

1 cup pitted dates

1 cup almonds

½ cup sweetened cocoa powder, plus extra for coating

½ cup unsweetened shredded coconut

¼ cup pure maple syrup

1 teaspoon vanilla extract

1 teaspoon almond extract

¼ teaspoon sea salt

Directions

1.   In the bowl of a food processor, combine all the ingredients and process until smooth. Chill the mixture for about 1 hour.

2.   Roll the mixture into balls and then roll the balls in cocoa powder to coat.

3.   Serve immediately or keep chilled until ready to serve.

Pecan and Date-Stuffed Roasted Pears

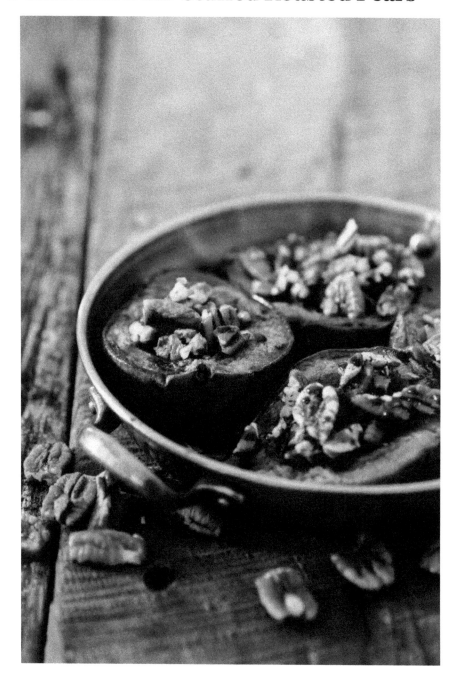

Preparation time: 10 minutes cooking time: 30 minutes servings: 4

Ingredients

4 firm ripe pears, cored

1 tablespoon fresh lemon juice

1/2 cup finely chopped pecans

4 dates, pitted and chopped

1 tablespoon vegan margarine

1 tablespoon pure maple syrup

1/4 teaspoon ground cinnamon

1/8 teaspoon ground ginger

1/2 cup pear, white grape, or apple juice

Directions

1.	Preheat the oven to 350°F. Grease a shallow baking dish and set aside. Halve the pears lengthwise and use a melon baller to scoop out the cores. Rub the exposed part of the pears with the lemon juice to avoid discoloration.

2.	In a medium bowl, combine the pecans, dates, margarine, maple syrup, cinnamon, and ginger and mix well.

3.	Stuff the mixture into the centers of the pear halves and arrange them in the prepared baking pan. Pour the juice over the pears. Bake until tender, 30 to 40 minutes. Serve warm.

Almond Balls

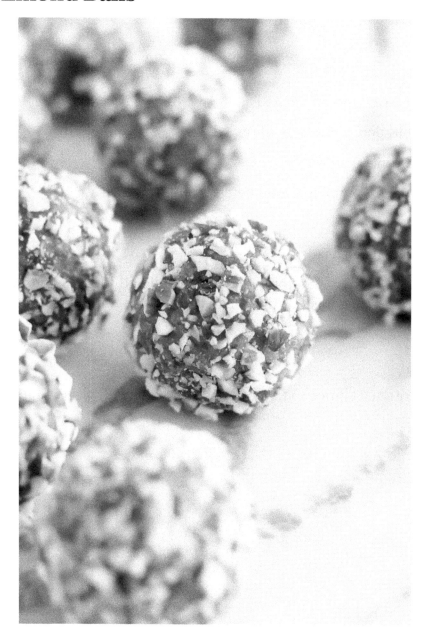

Preparation time: 10 minutes Cooking time: 0 minutes Servings: 6

Ingredients:

½ cup coconut oil, melted

5 tablespoons almonds, chopped

1 tablespoon stevia

¼ cup coconut flesh, unsweetened and shredded

Directions:

1.   In a bowl, combine the coconut oil with the almonds and the other ingredients, stir well and spoon into round moulds.

2.   Serve them cold.

Nutrition: calories 194, fat 21.2, fiber 0.7, carbs 1, protein 1.4

Grapefruit Cream

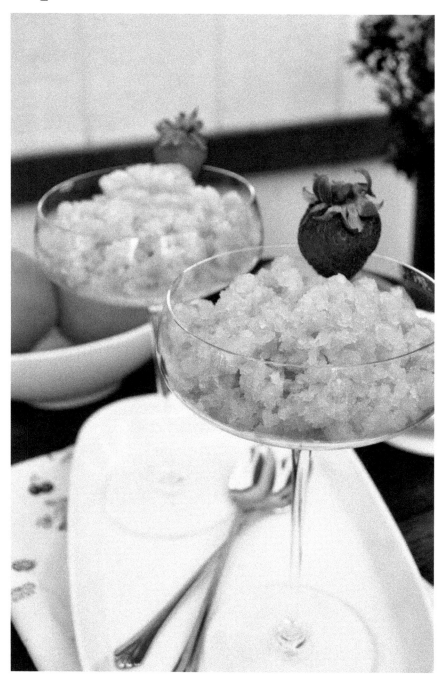

Preparation time: 10 minutes Cooking time: 0 minutes Servings: 4

Ingredients:

2 cups coconut cream

1 cup grapefruit, peeled, and chopped

2 tablespoons stevia

1 teaspoon vanilla extract

Directions:

1. In a blender, combine the coconut cream with the grapefruit and the other ingredients, pulse well, divide into bowls and serve cold.

Nutrition: calories 346, fat 35.5, fiber 0, carbs 3.4, protein 4.6

Tangerine Stew

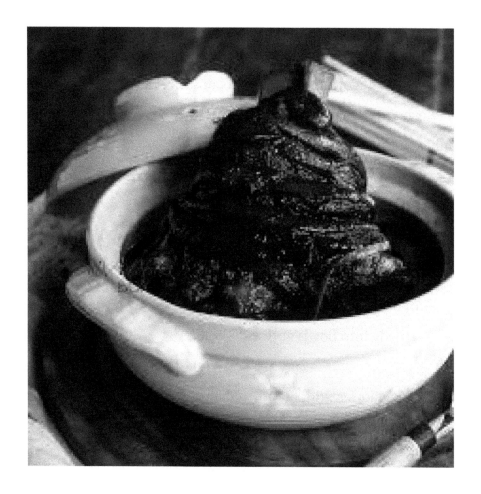

Preparation time: 10 minutes Cooking time: 10 minutes Servings: 4

Ingredients:

1   cup coconut water

2   cups tangerines, peeled and cut into segments

1 tablespoon lime juice

1 tablespoon stevia

½ teaspoon vanilla extract

Directions:

1.   In a pan, combine the coconut water with the tangerines and the other ingredients, toss, bring to a simmer and cook over medium heat for 10 minutes.

2.   Divide into bowls and serve cold.

Nutrition: calories 289, fat 26.1, fiber 3.9, carbs 10.3, protein 5.7

Creamy Pineapple Mix

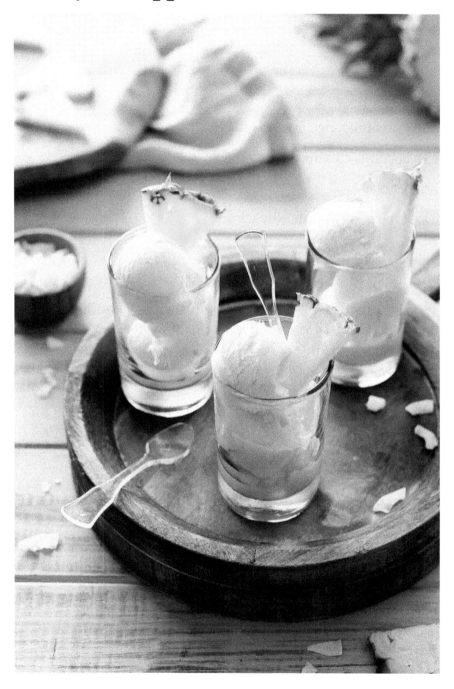

Preparation time: 10 minutes Cooking time: 10 minutes Servings: 4

Ingredients:

1 teaspoon nutmeg, ground

1 cup pineapple, peeled and cubed

1 cup coconut cream

½ cup stevia

1   teaspoon vanilla extract

Directions:

1.   In a pan, combine the pineapple with the nutmeg and the other ingredients, toss, cook over medium heat for 10 minutes, divide into bowls and serve.

Nutrition: calories 329, fat 32.7, fiber 0, carbs 2.5, protein 5.7

Avocado and Pineapple Bowls

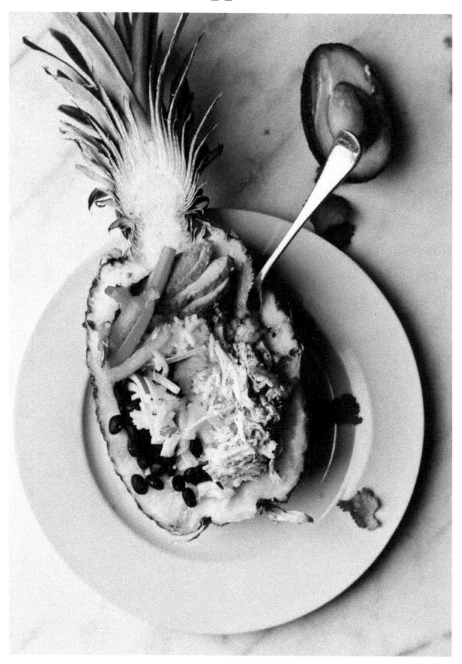

Preparation time: 10 minutes Cooking time: 0 minutes Servings: 4

Ingredients:

2   tablespoons avocado oil

1   cup pineapple, peeled and cubed

2   avocados, peeled, pitted and cubed 2 tablespoons stevia

Juice of 1 lime

Directions:

1.   In a bowl, combine the pineapple with the avocados and the other ingredients, toss, and serve cold.

Nutrition: calories 312, fat 29.5, fiber 3.3, carbs 16.7, protein 5

Pineapple and Melon Stew

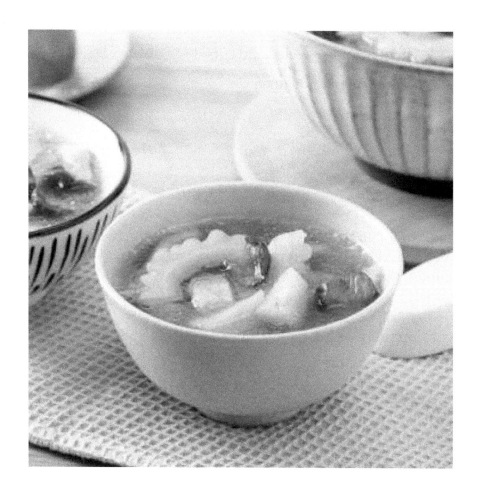

Preparation time: 10 minutes Cooking time: 15 minutes Servings: 4

Ingredients:

2 tablespoons stevia

1   cup pineapple, peeled and cubed

1 cup melon, peeled and cubed

2   cups water

1 teaspoon vanilla extract

Directions:

1.   In a pan, combine the pineapple with the melon and the other ingredients, toss gently, cook over medium-low heat for 15 minutes, divide into bowls and serve cold.

Nutrition: calories 40, fat 4.3, fiber 2.3, carbs 3.4, protein 0.8

Cocoa Muffins

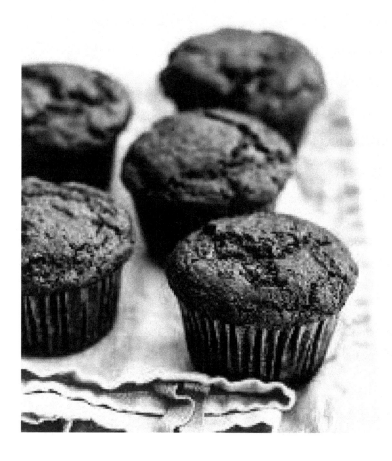

Preparation time: 10 minutes Cooking time: 25 minutes Servings: 6

Ingredients:

½ cup coconut oil, melted

3 tablespoons stevia

1 cup almond flour

¼ cup cocoa powder

3 tablespoons flaxseed mixed with

4 tablespoons water

¼ teaspoon vanilla extract

1 teaspoon baking powder Cooking spray

Directions:

1.   In bowl, combine the coconut oil with the stevia, the flour and the other ingredients except the cooking spray and whisk well.

2.   Grease a muffin pan with the cooking spray, divide the muffin mix in each mould, bake at 370 degrees F for 25 minutes, cool down and serve.

Nutrition: calories 344, fat 35.1, fiber 3.4, carbs 8.3, protein 4.5

Melon Coconut Mousse

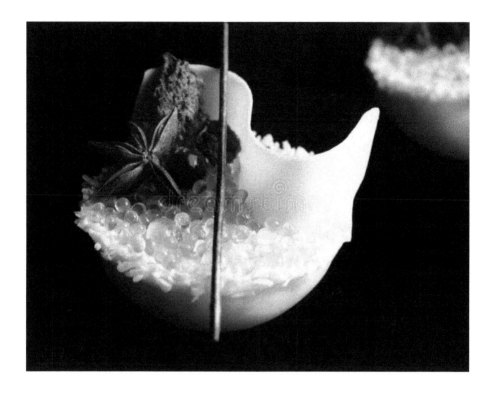

Preparation time: 10 minutes Cooking time: 0 minutes

Servings: 6

Ingredients:

2 cups coconut cream

1 teaspoon vanilla extract

1 tablespoon stevia

1 cup melon, peeled and chopped

Directions:

1. In a blender, combine the melon with the cream and the other ingredients, pulse well, divide into bowls and serve cold.

Nutrition: calories 219, fat 21.1, fiber 0.9, carbs 7, protein 1.4

Chia and Strawberries Mix

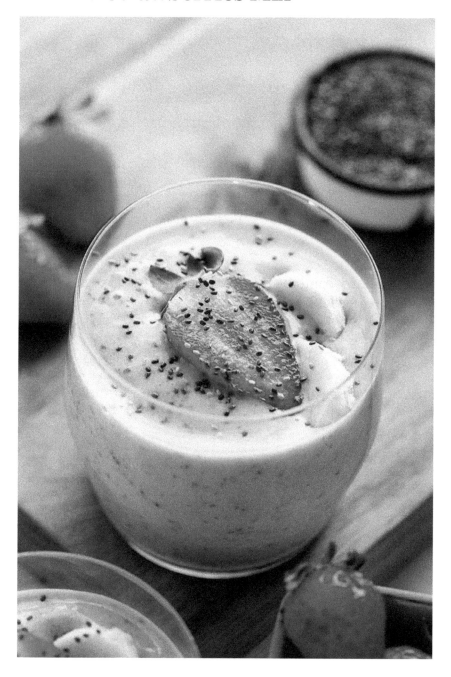

Preparation time: 10 minutes Cooking time: 0 minutes Servings: 4

Ingredients:

1 cup strawberries, halved

2 tablespoons chia seeds

¼ cup coconut milk

1 tablespoon stevia

Directions:

1.   In a bowl, combine the berries with the chia seeds, the milk and stevia and whisk well.

2.   Divide the mix into bowls and serve cold.

Nutrition: calories 265, fat 6.3, fiber 2, carbs 4, protein 6

Watermelon Mousse

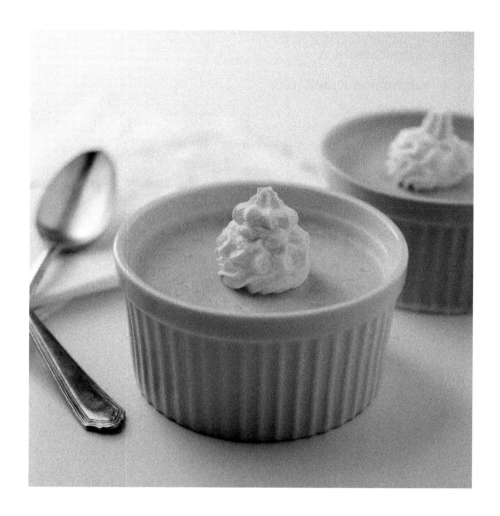

Preparation time: 10 minutes Cooking time: 0 minutes Servings: 4

Ingredients:

1 cup coconut cream

1   tablespoon lemon juice

1 tablespoon stevia

2   cups watermelon, peeled and cubed

Directions:

1.   In a blender, combine the watermelon with the cream, the lemon juice and stevia, pulse well, divide into bowls and serve cold.

Nutrition: calories 332, fat 31.4, fiber 0.5, carbs 9.2, protein 5.5

Fruit Salad

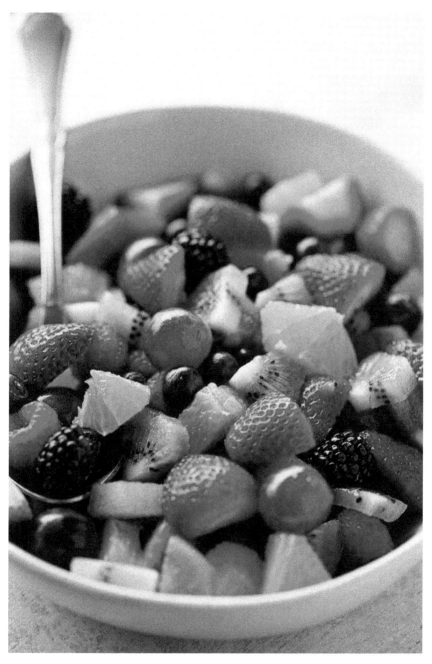

Preparation time: 2 hours Cooking time: 0 minutes Servings: 4

Ingredients:

2 avocados, peeled, pitted and cubed

½ cup blackberries

½ cup strawberries, halved

½ cup pineapple, peeled and cubed

¼ teaspoon vanilla extract

2 tablespoons stevia

Juice of 1 lime

Directions:

In a bowl, combine the avocados with the berries and the other ingredients, toss and keep in the fridge for 2 hours before serving.

Nutrition: calories 243, fat 22, fiber 0, carbs 6.2, protein 4

Chia Bars

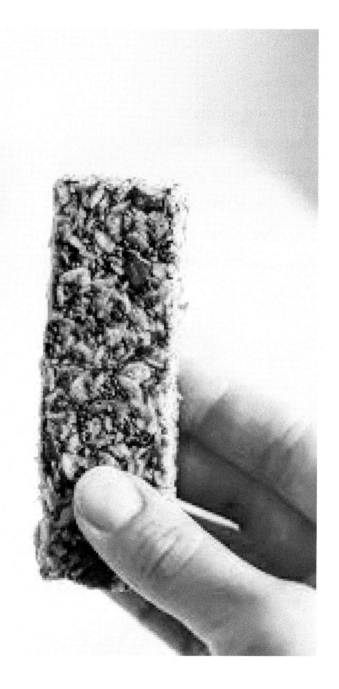

Preparation time: 10 minutes Cooking time: 20 minutes Servings: 6

Ingredients:

1 cup coconut oil, melted

½ teaspoon baking soda

3 tablespoons chia seeds

2 tablespoons stevia

1 cup coconut cream

3 tablespoons flaxseed mixed with

4 tablespoons water

Directions:

1.	In a bowl, combine the coconut oil with the cream, the chia seeds and the other ingredients, whisk well, pour everything into a square baking dish, introduce in the oven at 370 degrees F and bake for 20 minutes.

2.	Cool down, slice into squares and serve.

Nutrition: calories 220, fat 2, fiber 0.5, carbs 2, protein 4

Fruits Stew

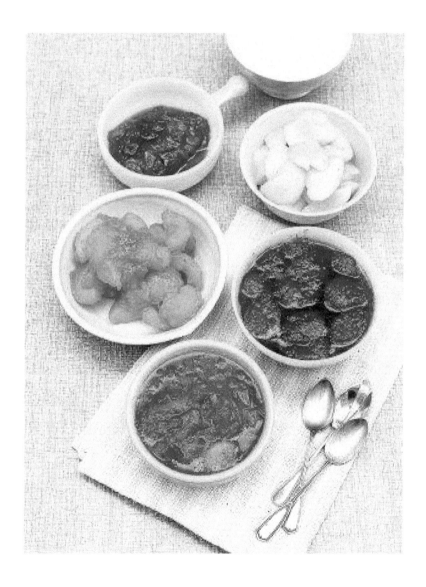

Preparation time: 10 minutes Cooking time: 10 minutes Servings: 4

Ingredients:

1   avocado, peeled, pitted and sliced

1 cup plums, stoned and halved

2   cups water

2 teaspoons vanilla extract

1 tablespoon lemon juice

2 tablespoons stevia

Directions:

1.   In a pan, combine the avocado with the plums, water and the other ingredients, bring to a simmer and cook over medium heat for 10 minutes.

2.   Divide the mix into bowls and serve cold.

Nutrition: calories 178, fat 4.4, fiber 2, carbs 3, protein 5

Avocado and Rhubarb Salad

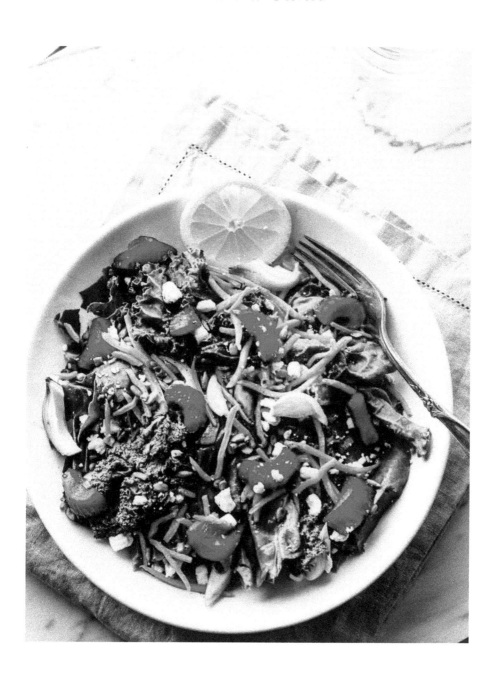

Preparation time: 10 minutes Cooking time: 0 minutes Servings: 4

Ingredients:

1 tablespoon stevia

1   cup rhubarb, sliced and boiled

2   avocados, peeled, pitted and sliced

1 teaspoon vanilla extract

Juice of 1 lime

Directions:

1.   In a bowl, combine the rhubarb with the avocado and the other ingredients, toss and serve.

Nutrition: calories 140, fat 2, fiber 2, carbs 4, protein 4

Plums and Nuts Bowls

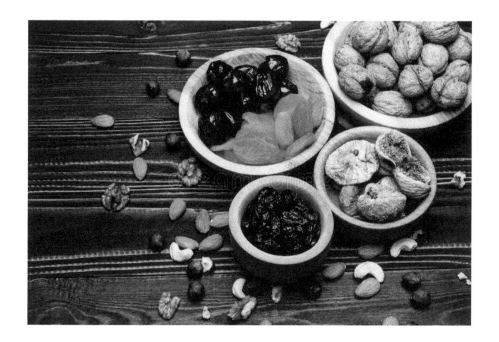

Preparation time: 5 minutes Cooking time: 0 minutes Servings: 2

Ingredients:

2 tablespoons stevia

1 cup walnuts, chopped

1   cup plums, pitted and halved

1 teaspoon vanilla extract

Directions:

1.   In a bowl, mix the plums with the walnuts and the other ingredients, toss, divide into 2 bowls and serve cold.

Nutrition: calories 400, fat 23, fiber 4, carbs 6, protein 7

Avocado and Strawberries Salad

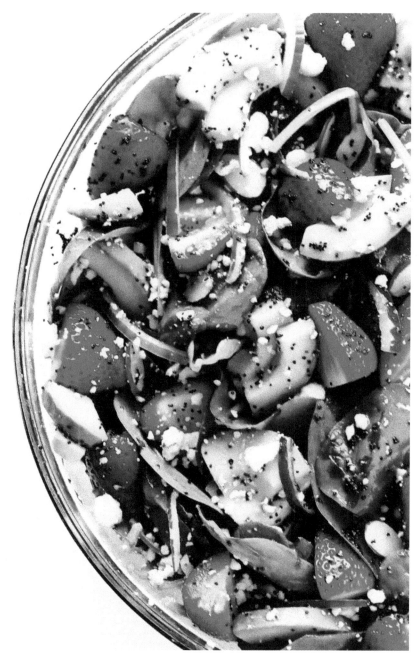

Preparation time: 5 minutes Cooking time: 0 minutes Servings: 4

Ingredients:

2   avocados, pitted, peeled and cubed

1 cup strawberries, halved

Juice of 1 lime

1   teaspoon almond extract

2   tablespoons almonds, chopped

1   tablespoon stevia

Directions:

1.   In a bowl, combine the avocados with the strawberries, and the other ingredients, toss and serve.

Nutrition: calories 150, fat 3, fiber 3, carbs 5, protein 6

Chocolate Watermelon Cups

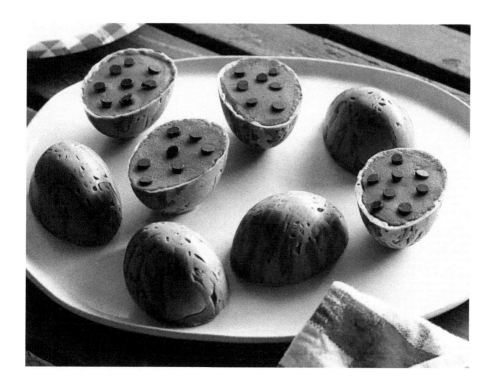

Preparation time: 2 hours Cooking time: 0 minutes Servings: 4

Ingredients:

2   cups watermelon, peeled and cubed

1 tablespoon stevia

1 cup coconut cream

1 tablespoon cocoa powder

1 tablespoon mint, chopped

Directions:

1.   In a blender, combine the watermelon with the stevia and the other ingredients, pulse well, divide into cups and keep in the fridge for 2 hours before serving.

Nutrition: calories 164, fat 14.6, fiber 2.1, carbs 9.9, protein 2.1

Vanilla Raspberries Mix

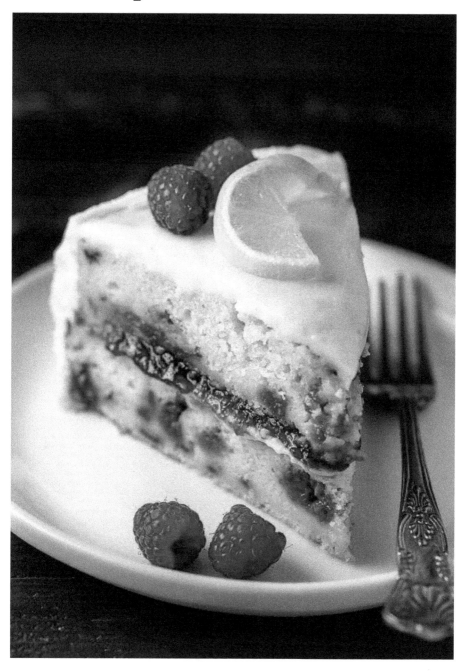

Preparation time: 10 minutes Cooking time: 10 minutes

Servings: 4

Ingredients:

1 cup water

1 cup raspberries

3 tablespoons stevia

1   teaspoon nutmeg, ground

½ teaspoon vanilla extract

Directions:

1.   In a pan, combine the raspberries with the water and the other ingredients, toss, cook over medium heat for 10 minutes, divide into bowls and serve.

Nutrition: calories 20, fat 0.4, fiber 2.1, carbs 4, protein 0.4

Ginger Cream

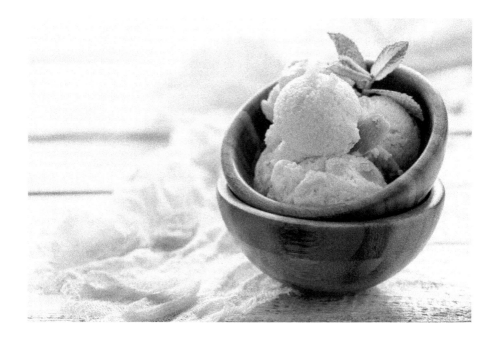

Preparation time: 10 minutes Cooking time: 10 minutes Servings: 4

Ingredients:

2   tablespoons stevia

2 cups coconut cream

1 teaspoon vanilla extract

1   tablespoon cinnamon powder

¼ tablespoon ginger, grated

Directions:

1.   In a pan, combine the cream with the stevia and other ingredients, stir, cook over medium heat for 10 minutes, divide into bowls and serve cold.

Nutrition: calories 280, fat 28.6, fiber 2.7, carbs 7, protein 2.8

Chocolate Ginger Cookies

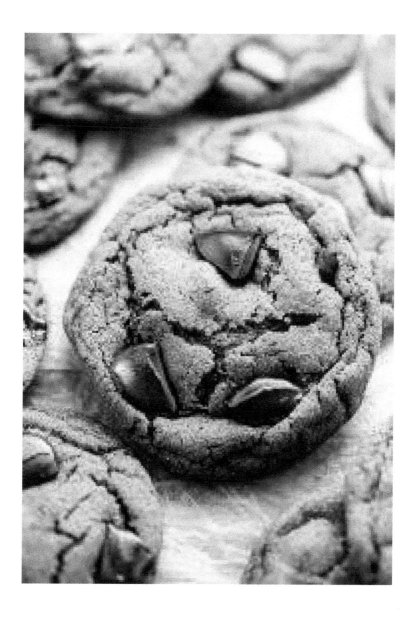

Preparation time: 10 minutes Cooking time: 20 minutes Servings: 6

Ingredients:

2   cups almonds, chopped

2 tablespoons flaxseed mixed with

3 tablespoons water

¼ cup avocado oil

2 tablespoons stevia

¼ cup cocoa powder

1   teaspoon baking soda

Directions:

1.   In your food processor, combine the almonds with the flaxseed mix and the other ingredients, pulse well, scoop tablespoons out of this mix, arrange them on a lined baking sheet, flatten them a bit and cook at 360 degrees F for 20 minutes.

2.   Serve the cookies cold.

Nutrition: calories 252, fat 41.6, fiber 6.5, carbs 11.7, protein 3

Coconut Salad

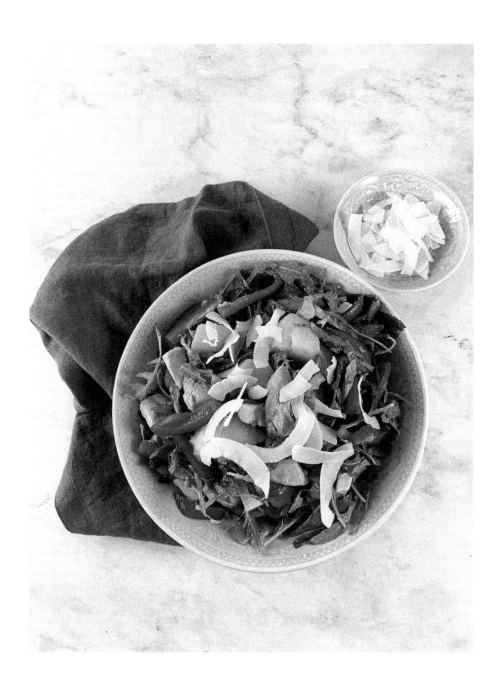

Preparation time: 10 minutes Cooking time: 0 minutes Servings: 6

Ingredients:

2   cups coconut flesh, unsweetened and shredded

½ cup walnuts, chopped

1 cup blackberries

1 tablespoon stevia

1   tablespoon coconut oil, melted

Directions:

1.   In a bowl, combine the coconut with the walnuts and the other ingredients, toss and serve.

Nutrition: calories 250, fat 23.8, fiber 5.8, carbs 8.9, protein 4.5

Mint Cookies

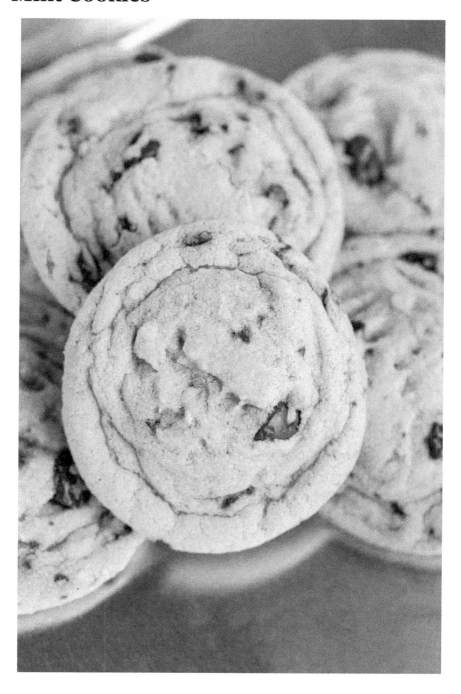

Preparation time: 10 minutes Cooking time: 20 minutes Servings: 6

Ingredients:

2   cups coconut flour

3   tablespoons flaxseed mixed with

4 tablespoons water

½ cup coconut cream

½ cup coconut oil, melted

3 tablespoons stevia

 2 teaspoons mint, dried

2 teaspoons baking soda

Directions:

1.   In a bowl, mix the coconut flour with the flaxseed, coconut cream and the other ingredients, and whisk really well.

2.   Shape balls out of this mix, place them on a lined baking sheet, flatten them, introduce in the oven at 370 degrees F and bake for 20 minutes.

3.   Serve the cookies cold.

Nutrition: calories 190, fat 7.32, fiber 2.2, carbs 4, protein 3

Mint Avocado Bars

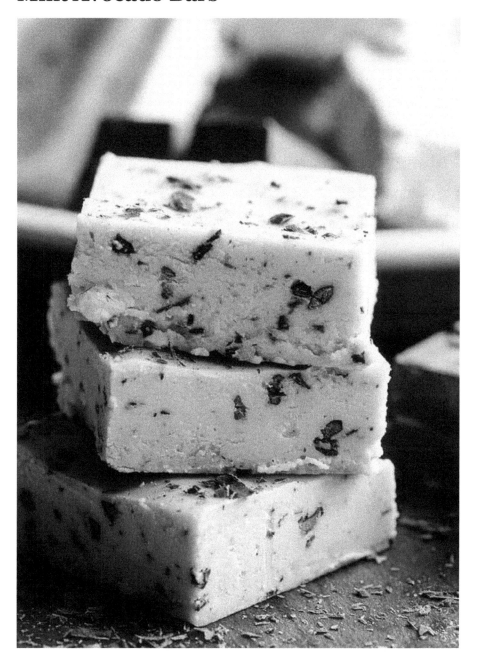

Preparation time: 10 minutes Cooking time: 25 minutes Servings: 6

Ingredients:

1 teaspoon almond extract

½ cup coconut oil, melted

2 tablespoons stevia

1 avocado, peeled, pitted and mashed

2 cups coconut flour

1 tablespoon cocoa powder

Directions:

1.   In a bowl, combine the coconut oil with the almond extract, stevia and the other ingredients and whisk well.

2.   Transfer this to baking pan, spread evenly, introduce in the oven and cook at 370 degrees F and bake for 25 minutes.

3.   Cool down, cut into bars and serve.

Nutrition: calories 230, fat 12.2, fiber 4.2, carbs 15.4, protein 5.8

Coconut Chocolate Cake

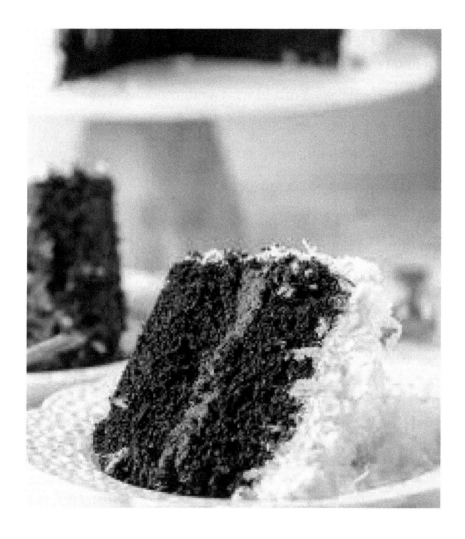

Preparation time: 10 minutes Cooking time: 30 minutes

Servings: 12

Ingredients:

4 tablespoons flaxseed mixed with 5 tablespoons water

1 cup coconut flesh, unsweetened and shredded

1   teaspoon vanilla extract

2   tablespoons cocoa powder

1 teaspoon baking soda

2 cups almond flour

4 tablespoons stevia

2 tablespoons lime zest

2 cups coconut cream

Directions:

1.   In a bowl, combine the flaxmeal with the coconut, the vanilla and the other ingredients, whisk well and transfer to a cake pan.

2.   Cook the cake at 360 degree F for 30 minutes, cool down and serve.

Nutrition: calories 268, fat 23.9, fiber 5.1, carbs 9.4, protein 6.1

Mint Chocolate Cream

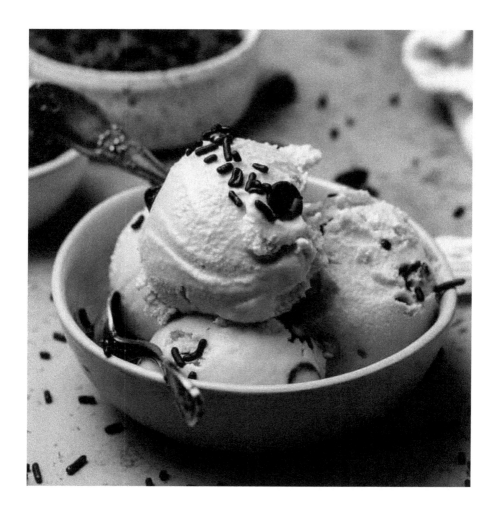

Preparation time: 10 minutes Cooking time: 0 minutes Servings: 6

Ingredients:

1 cup coconut oil, melted

4 tablespoons cocoa powder

1 teaspoon vanilla extract

1   cup mint, chopped

2 cups coconut cream

4 tablespoons stevia

Directions:

1.   In your food processor, combine the coconut oil with the cocoa powder, the cream and the other ingredients, pulse well, divide into bowls and serve really cold.

Nutrition: calories 514, fat 56, fiber 3.9, carbs 7.8, protein 3

Cranberries Cake

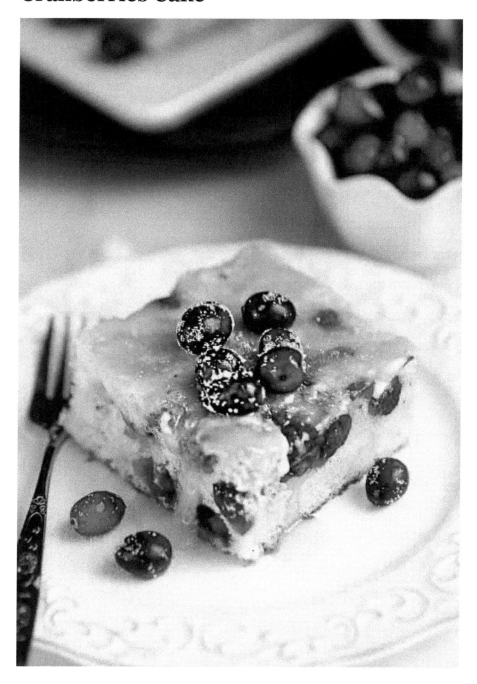

Preparation time: 10 minutes Cooking time: 30 minutes Servings: 6

Ingredients:

2   cups coconut flour

2 tablespoon coconut oil, melted

3 tablespoons stevia

1   tablespoon cocoa powder, unsweetened

2   tablespoons flaxseed mixed with

3 tablespoons water

1 cup cranberries

1 cup coconut cream

¼ teaspoon vanilla extract

½ teaspoon baking powder

Directions:

1.   In a bowl, combine the coconut flour with the coconut oil, the stevia and the other ingredients, and whisk well.

2.   Pour this into a cake pan lined with parchment paper, introduce in the oven and cook at 360 degrees F for 30 minutes.

3.   Cool down, slice and serve.

Nutrition: calories 244, fat 16.7, fiber 11.8, carbs 21.3, protein 4.4

Sweet Zucchini Buns

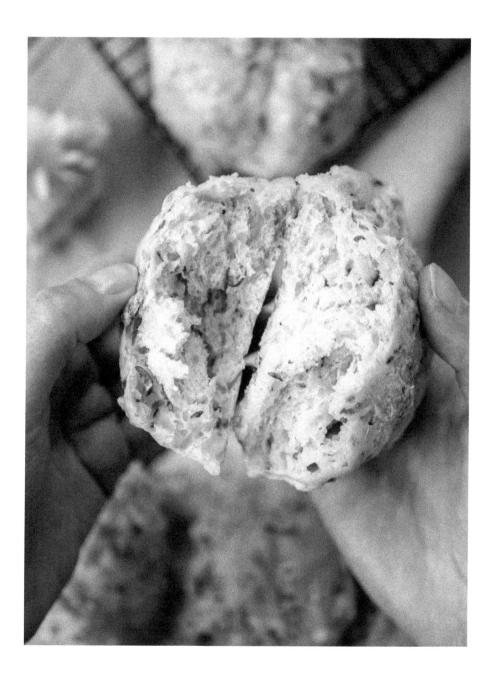

Preparation time: 10 minutes Cooking time: 30 minutes Servings: 8

Ingredients:

1   cup almond flour

1/3 cup coconut flesh, unsweetened and shredded

1 cup zucchinis, grated

2   tablespoons stevia

1 teaspoon baking soda

½ teaspoon cinnamon powder

3 tablespoons flaxseed mixed with

4 tablespoons water

1 cup coconut cream

Directions:

1.   In a bowl, mix the almond flour with the coconut flesh, the zucchinis and the other ingredients, stir well until you obtain a dough, shape 8 buns and arrange them on a baking sheet lined with parchment paper.

2.   Introduce in the oven at 350 degrees and bake for 30 minutes.

3.   Serve these sweet buns warm.

Nutrition: calories 169, fat 15.3, fiber 3.9, carbs 6.4, protein 3.2

Lime Custard

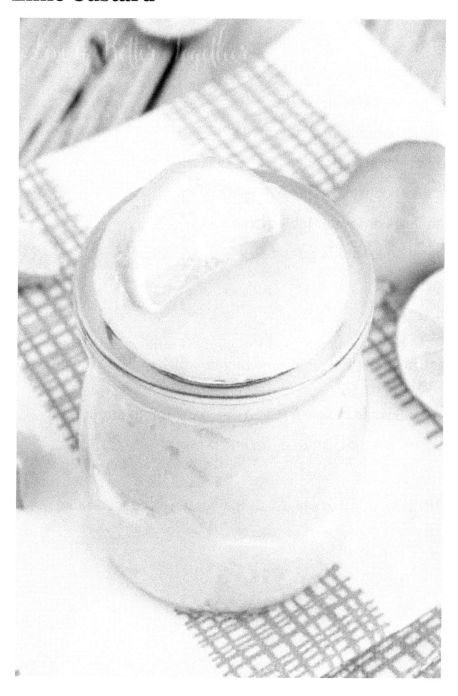

Preparation time: 10 minutes Cooking time: 20 minutes Servings: 6

Ingredients:

1 pint almond milk

4 tablespoons lime zest, grated

3 tablespoons lime juice

3 tablespoons flaxseed mixed with

4 tablespoons water tablespoons stevia

2 teaspoons vanilla extract

Directions:

1.   In a bowl, combine the almond milk with the lime zest, lime juice and the other ingredients, whisk well and divide into 4 ramekins.

2.   Bake in the oven at 360 degrees F for 30 minutes.

3.   Cool the custard down and serve.

Nutrition: calories 234, fat 21.6, fiber 4.3, carbs 9, protein 3.5

Lightning Source UK Ltd.
Milton Keynes UK
UKHW021015030521
383041UK00001B/92